HOW TO START A HOME HEALTH CARE AGENCY

HOW TO START A
HOME HEALTH
CARE AGENCY

Jeffie Maag
Owner & Operator of
XYZ Home Healthcare Services, LLC

Library of Congress Control Number:		2015901070
ISBN:	Hardcover	978-1-5035-3722-4
	Softcover	978-1-5035-3724-8
	eBook	978-1-5035-3723-1

Edited by Lilly Warren

Print information available on the last page.

Rev. date: 02/12/2015

To order additional copies of this book, contact:
Xlibris
1-888-795-4274
www.Xlibris.com
Orders@Xlibris.com
703717

CONTENTS

Dedicated To

I dedicate this book to my husband David, my son Donald, my daughter-in-law Angie, and Kim a close friend. They have all helped me make my dream a reality.

Most of all, I give thanks to GOD for giving me the confidence to venture out from my comfort zone and do something different.

CHAPTER 1

Introduction

As a young girl, I knew I wanted to grow up and make a difference in the lives of other people. What I had not planned on was the difference others would make in my life. My name is Jeffie and I am the owner of a "for profit" home health care agency which I started from the ground up. If given the opportunity to do things over in my life, I would change only one thing, and that would have been to start my own home health care agency years ago.

I began a life long adventure in the health care field starting as a nursing assistant, then becoming a licensed nurse and finally becoming an administrator in the long term care industry. I served as an administrator for nearly twenty three years before leaving. I was not ready to retire, yet I did not want to relocate to another city just to continue doing what I enjoyed doing.

For years I watched how other divisions of health care operated and was intrigued with the home health care area. Unlike the long term care industry where I was strong and knowledgeable, I had great difficulty piecing together information needed to open a home health care agency. I put months of hard work into researching and reading everything I could find. Once I had a good knowledge base for the home care industry, I talked things over with my family, and I knew I had their support and commitment to help me, so I decided to go for it.

Because of all the struggles I had, trying to get information on opening up a home health care agency, I decided that no one should have to go through all the trouble I did. It left me with no choice but to write this book. If your dream is to open a home health care agency, I know the information in this book will be very beneficial and I wish you the very best in your endeavor.

In this book I have included several forms that I developed for my agency, along with the Employee Handbook outline and Admission Booklet Contents. You may use them to help you develop your own booklets with written permission.

I do know you will benefit from this book immensely in helping you to open your own home health care agency. Each chapter may seem small but the actual work done to achieve the goal is great. Much of the information provided in this book is done simultaneously. I do not claim to have included all the steps in this book that may be necessary, and requirements will vary from state to state.

The information in this book will help you to open any type of home health agency, it all depends on what type of home health agency you want. I chose to deal with children because that was where my heart was. I do not recommend trying to take care of all age groups and all insurance coverage types when you first start out because it can get very confusing.

No matter what you decide on just be sure to document your actions on a daily basis, especially who you talk with and what you discussed. Keep all documentation in a binder so you can find it easily when needed.

CHAPTER 2

Is This Right For You?

Even with all the stumbling blocks I encountered, I knew that being a home health care agency owner was what I was going to do. I had limited resources and lacked recent experience as a hands-on nurse. Both proved to be a big challenge for me. All I knew was that I was going for it or fall hard trying. So no matter what your situation, if this is something you really want, go for it, but be willing to put in the time to achieve it.

In starting a home health care agency it is advisable that you are a nurse or have good administrative experience in the health care field because of all the State Regulations and Federal Rules and Regulations that must be followed. If you are not a nurse then you need to consider contracting with an RN to help you in the nursing areas.

There is a step by step process one must follow and it takes months to get to a point where your agency is ready for survey. There are certain guidelines set by your state and the federal government which you will have no control over but must follow.

Allow six to eight months to get your policies, staff and clients ready before asking for a Probationary License, which is necessary for you to open the doors to your home health care agency.

Once you have your Probationary License you have six months to demonstrate that you know what you are doing. During this time your state will conduct an initial survey to determine if you are in compliance with state and federal guidelines regarding home health care. You would think by now you would be ready to start taking on paying clients, but unless you are fortunate enough to get all private pay clients you will need to apply for your state funded programs following your initial survey. This can take two to four months to work through all the red tape. Just keep in mind, the end results are well worth all the trouble and waiting you go through.

Remember to document any and all actions taken. I highly recommend you get a 5 inch binder to keep notes and applications in. It is easy to drown in the paper work if you are not organized to start with.

CHAPTER 3

Getting Prepared

Getting prepared means having dedicated space for an office. I started my agency in my own home. Because of the amount of time involved to get the business started, I could not afford to rent a business location, so I converted half of my living room into office space and it has worked out well for me. Check with your local zoning board to make sure you can start a home based business in your home.

As with any business you will need certain items to help you get the job done. Even though some of the items listed will not be used until a later date, you need to go ahead and have them on hand.

Items Needed:

Computer	Printer
Removable Disk	Internet
Dedicated Telephone Line & Number	
Dedicated Fax Line & Number	
E-Mail Address	Web Site
Desk & Chair	Filing Cabinet
File Folders	Copy Paper
Computerized Office Accounting System	Dictionary
Calculator	Rolodex

Jeffie Maag

Binders 4" to 5"   Shredder
Hole Puncher   Stapler
Paper Clips   White Out
Envelopes   Letter Head
Stamps
Pens, mainly black with several blue and red
Pencils
Pencil Sharpener

CHAPTER 4

Who Are My Clients?

Before naming your agency you need to decide on whom you want as your clients. Do you want to deal with a certain age group, such as children, the disabled, or the aged? Do you want to be an agency that goes in the home and performs specified tasks once or twice a week, or do you want to take care of clients requiring up to 12 hours a day skilled nursing coverage?

Children may require up to 24 hours a day coverage for medically complex needs, whereas the disabled and aged individuals may only require an hour on a daily basis or possibly up to four hours 2 to 4 times a week.

When making your decision, take into consideration the census for your selected area. Also, take into consideration the availability of nurses and home health aides for your selected area.

For my home health care agency, I chose to care for children and young adults with medically complex needs. These agencies are in great demand for the area we serve. Another reason for choosing to work with children is that reimbursement is funded through Medicaid (state funding).

Now that you know whom your client base is going to be, start working on your agency name. This should be catchy enough to get people's attention. Keep in mind that you need to end the company name with Home Health Care Agency to prevent any confusion as to what type of business you are. I did not follow this advise and sometimes people get confused as to what type of service my agency provides. I chose Pediatric Plus Home Healthcare Services as my company name. Pediatrics tells people that we care for children, and to cover all bases I added in the Plus to cover individuals over the age of 21, just in case we decided to take someone older.

As a preliminary measure, once you decide on the name for your agency, go online and see if there is another agency in your state with the same name. If the name for your agency is not already in use, you should contact the Secretary of State to find out what you need to do to reserve the name for your agency. There is a fee involved with this step.

CHAPTER 5

Getting Started

Contact your state's department of health to find out what is required to open a home health care agency. You will need to apply for a National Provider Number, which is discussed in Chapter 9 before registering your business with the Secretary of State. You can go online to the Secretary of State web site and get the information you need to start up a business, and an outline is provided on Choosing a Structure and Forming Your Business.

It is advisable to talk with a tax accountant or attorney on which type of structure you should organize under. Keep in mind that no matter what structure you form your business under, you will be taxed.

An important factor to remember is that once you register your business, you don't want to change it. When you submit your applications to the various organizations you do not want to have to redo those applications any time soon.

I made the mistake of not consulting with a tax expert and found myself being taxed heavily. I have since changed my business to an S Corporation and added my son as co-owner in the event something should happen to me. So PLEASE, put plenty of thought into this matter before doing anything.

Once you have determined which structure you want for your business, go ahead and develop your company brochure, Business Plan and By-Laws.

I also recommend that if you have the money, join your state Home Health Care Association. This organization is a great resource which keeps you updated on changes related to state and federal regulations.

CHAPTER 6

Brochure Development

Now that you know what type of clients you want to care for, you need to start working on what you want your company brochure to say.

Our brochure is a tri-fold. The first section is the Welcome statement which tells a person a little about our company, types of services we provide, and types of payer sources we accept.

The middle section is all about the history of how our agency came about. It also includes information on myself and my son, the owners and operators of the agency. Keep in mind that most people like to know who you are and if you are local, or from some other state.

The next section contains our Mission Statement, our Vision Statement, and Our Values. When developing this section of the brochure, take plenty of time to make it impressive. Believe it or not, people like knowing as much as possible about a company that is asking for their business. Many times a brochure can make or break your business and the same goes for your business cards. Something just thrown together comes across as a questionable business, but when plenty of thought has gone into your brochure and business card, it shows.

The front of the brochure should be eye appealing so people will want to pick it up. Think about what colors you want to use and ask yourself if the colors and design reflect your agency.

Brochures look best when printed on a quality stock specifically for brochures. I suggest you only print what you will need for a few months. Without doubt you will want to make some changes later.

It took me almost a year and a half to finalize my brochure. Because there is so much to do in the beginning you will most likely miss some of the details of what it is you really want to say and project to potential clients.

A quality brochure makes it a little easler to develop a great web page, and a web page is a requirement in my state and most likely a requirement in other states as well.

By no means was my original brochure what I ended up with, but it helped me to keep my dream alive throughout the entire process of getting my agency up and running. Perhaps the best thing about your brochure is that it will be something you can look at when you are ready to throw in the towel. So let your brochure keep your dream alive.

CHAPTER 7

Business Plan

Regardless of the type of business or the size of the business, it is advisable to develop a business plan. This will help you stay focused and give you some direction.

According to the Small Business Administration, a business plan consist of 5 key areas:

1. The business plan should tell a compelling story about your business, explaining who, what, when, where, how and why.
2. Your plan should be focused and clear.
3. The plan should define specific business objectives and goals with general parameters to guide the organization.
4. Writing a business plan should force logic and discipline into a business.
5. A good business plan is a living document. It should be updated regularly.

A Business Plan needs to be a working tool, not a work of art. The Small Business Administration has a web site which has a template to help you build your business plan.

Jeffie Maag

The site I found to be user friendly was www.web.sba.gov/busplantemplate/BizPlanStart.cfm. Whether you choose to use this web site or another makes no difference, but developing a business plan is very important to the success of your business venture.

Once you have developed your business plan, put it in a place where you can refer back to it on a regular basis. A business plan helps to keep you motivated to stay on target.

A formal business plan is required if you should seek funding from an individual or lending institution.

CHAPTER 8

By-Laws

The next thing you will need to do is to decide if you are going to be the sole owner of your agency or have partners. Making this decision up front makes it easier to write by-laws for your agency's operation. By-Laws are required when registering your agency with the Secretary of State.

I went online and searched for various types and templates for by-laws. There are a lot of FREE templates for Limited Liability Companies as well as Corporations.

As a sole owner you can most likely write your own By-Laws; however, if you are uncomfortable writing By-Laws or if you are going to register your agency as a corporation, consider hiring a local attorney to help you develop your By-Laws. For a Limited Liability Company the term used for by-laws is Operating Agreement. There are several companies on the internet that perform this service as well.

By-Laws or Operating Agreement consist of 7 areas:

    ARTICLE 1 - Company Formation
    ARTICLE 2 - Capital Contributions
    ARTICLE 3 - Profits, Losses and Distributions
    ARTICLE 4 - Management

Jeffie Maag

ARTICLE 5 - Compensation
ARTICLE 6 - Bookkeeping
ARTICLE 7 - Transfers

During the start up process of your agency, review your by-laws on a regular basis and update as needed.

CHAPTER 9

National Provider Number

Before being able to register your agency with the Secretary of State you will need to have a National Provider Number. This application must be completed by, or on behalf of, a health care provider seeking to obtain an NPI.

You can retrieve this application from the internet. Because a National Provider Number is linked to the medical field, you can go to your State Department of Health web-site and possibly locate the application under the HIPAA Compliance section or use the follow information:

NPI Enumerator Contact Information:

By Phone: 1-800-465-3203
By E-mail: customerservice@npienumerator.com
By Mail: NPI Enumerator
             PO Box 6059
             Fargo, ND 58108-6059

Information required to complete the application consist of:

SECTION 1 - BASIC INFORMATION

    A.   Reason for Submittal of the Form
    B.   Entity Type

SECTION 2 - IDENTIFYING INFORMATION

    A. Individual Information
    B. Organization Information

SECTION 3 - ADDRESSES AND OTHER INFORMATION

    A.   Business Mailing Address Information
    B.   Business Practice Location Information
    C.   Other Provider Identification Numbers
    D.   Provider Taxonomy Code

Information on Taxonomy Codes is available at www.edi.com/taxonomy. For Home Health the Primary Taxonomy Code is 251E00 000X.

SECTION 4 - CERTIFICATION STATEMENT

Authorized Official's Information and Signature for the Organization.

SECTION 5 - CONTACT PERSON

The contact person should be the owner and should be readily available if called.

Print off the NPI form and directions. Read the directions and follow them to the letter. The form may appear intimidating at first but once you fill in the blanks as directed you will see that it is basic information being requested. On the form you will be submitting, I recommend you type in the answers instead of writing them in by hand.

CHAPTER 10

Uncle Sam Wants In

We all know that where there is money there are taxes, and no business can operate without having tax identification numbers. Even though you will not be fully operational for many months, you need to start the process to get your tax numbers. The good thing is that you are able to put an anticipated start date on the form. You will need your tax numbers for most of the applications you will be submitting.

You will need to complete a Business License Application to operate within your state. This process will provide you with your State Withholding Number and Unemployment Tax Number. I suggest you visit your local State Department of Revenue and they will provide you with the appropriate form. Be sure to keep a copy of this form in the binder.

The State Department of Revenue will send you your State Withholding Tax number and additional information you will need to provide to the company that will be doing your payroll.

Another tax identification number you will apply for is your Employer Identification Number (EIN). You can get the application at www.irs.gov. Keep a copy of this form in the binder. You will receive a letter once you have been assigned your Employer Identification Number. Be sure to keep the original document in a safe place since it is only issued one time and the IRS will not be able to generate a duplicate copy for you.

If you are uncomfortable doing these tax forms, contact your local tax accountant and he/she will assist you.

Be sure to allow yourself adequate time in projecting the Start of Business date. I allowed myself eight months.

As an employer you are responsible to post Required Employer Posters. State Posters can be obtained through your local Department of Revenue and Federal Posters can be purchased at your local office supply store. For more information about poster requirements or other compliance assistance matters, contact the U.S. Department of Labor by phone at 1-888-972-7332 or visit the DOL Poster Page.

CHAPTER 11

Web Page

By now you have developed your brochure. A brochure can be as simple or as elaborate as you want it, and should be used to help design your web page. Keep in mind that there is a cost involved with this process even if you do it all yourself.

Use your brochure to develop you Web Page. A brochure is a great marketing tool when presented well, and I recommend your Web Page be as similar to your brochure as possible. Tell what services you offer, a little about who owns and operates the agency, how someone can apply for a job with your agency, your address, phone number, and any other information you want to share. A picture of yourself is always a good idea.

A Web Page is required in most states for a home health care agency. Even if your state does not require you to have a web site, it just makes good business sense to have one. More and more people go to the internet to locate a service they need. You do not need a real elaborate Web Page, you just need a nice looking and informative Web Page.

There are several companies on the internet that will set up your Web Page and web site. Look for a company that is not real expensive.

CHAPTER 12

Registering Your Home Health Agency

Now that you have reserved the agency name with the Secretary of State, obtained a National Provider Number, developed By-Laws, have your tax numbers and a Web Site, you are ready to register your home health care agency.

Most states have the appropriate form available on the internet to register a new business with the Secretary of State. Most states require the same information, which is:

- Name of the business
- Address of the business
- Telephone number of the business
- National Provider Number assigned to the business
- Name of the Managing individuals
- Percent of ownership

The form is easy to fill out and will require a fee when you send it in. Keep a copy of the form in the binder.

Within a few weeks you will receive an official copy of where your business was registered with the Secretary of State. There will be two pages and it is very important to keep them together. Place a copy in the binder and frame the original and place it on the office wall.

Every two years you will be required to submit a report to the Secretary of State.

CHAPTER 13

CLIA Waiver

A CLIA Waiver is required for medical providers, and home health care is no exception.

To apply for a CLIA Waiver go to Centers for Medicare and Medicaid Services at www.cms.hhs.gov/clia to print off the application (CMS-116 form) and instructions. To determine where to send the CLIA Waiver Application once completed, click on the State Agency and Regional Office CLIA Contact section on the left side of the page. Look up your state to get the address and contact information needed.

This application is used for all laboratories and is full of questions, so remember to read the directions and complete only the sections required for your business. Should you have questions, you can call the Director of Home Health Care at your state level to help you. While you are on the CMS web page go ahead and locate the brochure called Clinical Laboratory Improvement Amendments (CLIA) Complaints and print it off. You will need this to give to clients that have lab work performed by your agency.

There is a fee required when filing for a CLIA Waiver.

Be sure to keep a copy of the application in your binder, and once you receive the official CLIA Waiver Certificate, make a copy of it to put in your binder and frame the original version and place on the office wall.

CHAPTER 14

Policy Development

Policy development is a very time consuming process if you do them all yourself. I had a lot of experience in policy development but due to my inexperience in the home health care industry, I had to research a number of online companies. I found one that had most of what I needed. Even though the cost involved seemed high, trust me, it was well worth the product I received. The internet company I used was MCN Policy Library of Healthcare Policies and Procedures and the web site is www.mcnhealthcare.com/.

If you are familiar with the Federal Rules and Regulations for Home Health Care Agencies, you can develop your own policies from them. To obtain a copy of the Federal Rules and Regulations, contact your State Department of Health and ask for the Home Health Agency Director. He/she will be able to tell you how to access the appropriate Federal Rules and Regulations, as well as your State Rules and Regulations if applicable. Be sure to write everything down exactly as it is given to you. There is a letter assigned to each tag number and may vary from state to state. Be sure to get the correct set of Federal Rules and Regulations for your state. Not all states have their own rules and regulations and only use the Federal Rules and Regulations.

Jeffie Maag

Even though this chapter is short, I must warn you that this is the most time consuming of all the processes you will do. For nursing policies and procedures I bought a number of nursing books that covered most nursing standards of practice.

CHAPTER 15

Employee Handbook

I am a firm believer that if you are wanting to project a professional image, then you need to do things in a professional manner. To save money and still be able to project a professional image, I purchased a book binding machine so that I could bind my Employee Handbook.

Keep in mind that your employees are your customers, in addition to the clients you will be taking care of. Avoid running copies from copies. Before you know it, the printed materials that you hand out will be of poor quality, so keep an original set of information available to copy from or have the information in your computer so you can run off copies as you need them.

Employee handbooks can include as much or as little information as you choose to put in them. I have a tendency to go overboard because I do not like dealing with loose papers. They are just too easy to misplace.

In the federal regulations there are certain areas that you must cover with all new hires. I believe each of these areas is covered in my Employee Handbook; however, as new requirements are mandated on a regular basis, your handbook should be updated to reflect them.

The following is the information I used in my original Employee Handbook:

- Welcome Statement
- Company History
- Mission Statement, Company Vision, Company Values and Philosophy
- Roles and Responsibilities of Interdisciplinary Healthcare Team
- Telephone Listings
- Accommodations for Disabilities
- Types of Care and Services Provided
- Ethics
- Personnel Policies
- Confidentiality of Patient, Staff & Organizational Information
- All Forms of Harassment
- Introductory Period
- Drug Free Work Place
- Employee Status
- Employee Conduct
- Attendance
- Employee Illness
- Picture Identification
- Appearance/Dress Code
- Gifts
- Scheduled Hours
- Overtime
- Meals and Breaks
- Holiday's/Sick Time
- Pay Check Distribution
- Insurance
- Educational Training
- Non-Competition Agreement
- Ethical Dilemmas In Patient Care
- Allegations of Theft
- Disciplinary Process
- General Procedures Involving Disciplinary Action
- Garnishment of Wages

- Employee Grievance Reporting Process
- Solicitation and Distribution
- Personnel Files
- Company Property
- Exit Interviews
- Hand Hygiene
- Back Safety and Body Mechanics
- Accident and Incident Reporting
- Fire Safety at Home Office and Client's Home
- Confidentiality/HIPAA
- Patient Rights and Responsibilities
- Advance Directives/Living Wills
- Death and Dying
- Patient Abuse
- Bureau of Developmental Disabilities Incident Reporting
- Conclusion

All employees must take a comprehensive post-test after completing general orientation. This helps us to understand their level of comprehension and their understanding of what is expected of them while in our employment.

CHAPTER 16

Annual In-Services

When distribution of new information or training is required, it is done as an in-service. If the information is required to be presented to employees on an annual basis, I include it in the Employee Handbook. Yearly, my employees are re-educated on the Employee Handbook which includes any new information.

As you are developing your Employee Handbook and Policies, it is a good time to go ahead and work with the RN to develop your annual in-service calendar. Set up an inservice binder and as you are reading a policy that is to be reviewed with your employees on an annual basis, make a copy of it and place it in the In-Service Binder. Once all the information is in the binder, the RN can set up the calendar and develop the post-test for each in-service. My company requires each employee to have at least one hour of in-service education monthly. To save time and to help my company stay in compliance, I purchased a number of educational materials from Beta Channing Company.

In the In-Service binder, we keep a copy of the annual In-Service Calendar with all the in-service material in month order. With each in-service we attach a copy of the Post-Test. Once the employee has taken a test and passed, it is filed in his/her employee folder. The majority of our in-service material is handed out at the first of the month with pay stubs and the employee is responsible for reading the information, taking the test and getting it back to the office by the 15th of each month. Some in-services are done face-to-face, and some are conducted by outside vendors.

Know what your state requirements are for in-service education for nurses and home health aides. Investing in your employees educational training is an excellent way for them to know what is expected of them at all times.

An example of an Annual In-Service Calendar is as follows:

ANNUAL IN-SERVICE CALENDAR
For All Staff
20_____

January: Topic
Infection Control, Hand- washing, Blood Borne Pathogens
February: Topic
HIPAA and Confidentially
March: Topic

There may be times when you have to conduct an in-service on a topic not listed on your annual calendar; be sure to write it in on the calendar and take credit for it.

CHAPTER 17

Lining Up Your Key Staff

I was fortunate to have a son and daughter-in-law and a close friend with whom I shared my desire to open a home health care agency. I needed them to help me and to serve in specific capacities within my organization. To my relief they all agreed to help me out. I knew this was an important step. My key staff had to go through the New Hire Information Process outlined in Chapter 18 before I could move forward.

When you make an application request from your State Department of Health you will need to list all your key people. Someone has to be appointed as the Administrator and a back-up administrator is required. For the Director of Clinical Services you must have an RN with management experience and a back-up RN for this position as well.

The above individuals will need to have a detailed resume with emphasis on their management and/or nursing experience. A copy of the tuberculin skin test (PPD), physical, professional license, and a Criminal Check as required by state.

You are now one step closer to being ready to submit your Probationary License Application to your State Department of Health.

CHAPTER 18

New Hire Information

Even though the agency has yet to generate any business, you will need to get your key people in place and there is no exception when it comes to the paperwork required for new hires. In this chapter I will share with you what I believe to be an easy and efficient way to stay organized when it comes to meeting the requirements for new hires.

There are three areas to cover for new hires and they are broken down by area.

Area 1: Pre-Employment Process

Employment Applications can be purchased from your local office supply store. Review the application for completeness, signature and date.

Ask the applicant for a copy of his/her resume.

Obtain two professional reference checks on potential new hires. If the individual lacks experience or has only held one position, design your policies to allow you to obtain a personal reference as needed.

Area 2: Hiring Process

A pre-employment physical and initial PPD is required. In the healthcare setting, and employees are also required to have a 2nd step PPD. Be sure to follow your state guidelines for PPD requirements.

I made arrangements with a local Nurse Practitioner to provide pre-employment physicals and PPD's to all potential new hires at a reasonable cost since my agency pays for this service.

You will need to make a copy from the originals of the following:

- Driver's License
- Social Security Card
- Professional License
- CPR & First Aid Card
- Auto Insurance Card

Complete a Rate of Pay Agreement with both the potential new hire and employer's signatures. By completing this form prevents any misunderstanding later on.

Individuals you intent to hire will need to have a Limited Criminal Check done. This process is required by most states and your State Department of Health will provide you with their specific requirements and the web site you will need to use. There is a cost associated with this process. While doing a limited criminal check go ahead and do a MVA check on every potential new hire.

Keep in mind that a potential new hire must meet all these standards before being given a hire date.

Area 3: General Orientation

The day of General Orientation is considered the hire date and the employee will need to complete the following:
- State With-holding Tax Form. You can pick this form up at your local State Department of Revenue or obtain it online.

- Federal With-holding Tax Form. You can obtain this form online by typing in "IRS FORMS" and it will take you to Forms and Publications Internal Revenue Services. Click on "Find a copy" of any necessary form. A list will come up and you can type in the Find Section "W-4" and hit search. The W-4 form is titled Employee's Withholding Allowance Certificate. Click on it and then print the form. Have the new hire complete this form, sign and date.

- I-9 Form. The I-9 Form can be printed off the internet. Go to Department of Homeland Security and click on Form I-9 Employment Eligibility Verification. Download and print the form. Be sure to read the form and all instructions. The new hire will complete the top section and the employer will complete the remaining sections.

- Review the job description with the new hire. Be sure it is signed and dated.

Now you are finally ready to conduct General Orientation. An RN will need to conduct a Skills Check List and schedule the employee for Client Specific Orientation before assigning the nurse or home health aide to care for the client independently.

There are a lot of requirements that must be met when hiring staff and it is easy to find your agency is in a non-compliant state if you do not have quality systems in place to keep your agency compliant with state and federal requirements.

Developing a Tracking System is an excellent way to help you stay organized. Employees and potential employees can be your biggest asset to the agency. Everyone that applies for a position with your agency should be treated with courtesy and respect, whether you hire them or not. I am a firm believer that anyone applying for a position should leave our agency with the attitude that we are the employer of choice, whether or not they become a team member. To help us track incoming information for potential new hires, we use the following layout:

New Hire Applicant Tracking Form

Name

Resume

Application Complete

Position Applied For

Reference Checks Done

Interview Schedule Date

Potential Hire Date

Rate of Pay Agreement

Pre-Employment Physical

1st Step PPD

Given & Read

Date Scheduled for 2nd Step PPD

Copy of Professional License & Verification

Copy of CPR & First Aid

Criminal Check Done

Date For General Orientation

Motor Vehicle Check Done

State and Federal Tax Forms Completed

Job Description Signed

General Orientation Post-test completed

Skills Check-List Completed

Client Specific Orientation Form Completed

I-9 Completed

The I-9 form is to be kept in a binder in alphabetic order and kept under lock and key.

CHAPTER 19

General Orientation For New Hires

You can tell new hires everything they need to know, but if there is not some form of documentation with the new hires' signature on it, you will run into problems, not only with the state during your initial survey, but with other governmental agencies as well.

For each Employee Handbook we printed, we added an Acknowledgment Form and Post-Test on the information presented in order to determine the new hires level of understanding. These papers then become a part of the employees permanent file.

CHAPTER 20

Job Descriptions

No matter what position a person holds within your agency, a Job Description must be reviewed, signed and placed in the employee file.

The job descriptions I use were purchased through MCN Library and they are very comprehensive. If you have the time, you can develop your own Job Descriptions. However, it is very time consuming.

The main thing is to have a Job Description for each position, review it with the new hire, and have him/her sign and date it. When employees know what is expected of them in their job roles, it makes it easier for you as the employer to hold your employees accountable.

CHAPTER 21

Employee Competency Skills Checklist

Employee Competency Skills Checklist were included in with the Job Descriptions purchased through MCN Library. Competency Skills Checklist were done on all of my key staff. This process allows management to know exactly what a person knows and where a person needs additional training. Additionally, Age Related Competency Checklist were completed on each nursing staff member as well.

Keep in mind that this process is required and forms are to be kept in the employee file and will be reviewed during the initial survey process by your state.

CHAPTER 22

Admission Booklet

Once again, I wanted to make sure my agency presented a professional image and I developed the Admission paper work and made it into a booklet.

Since much of the information used in the admission process is required and in some cases provided by government agencies, I included it in the Admission Booklet along with all the specific information we use.

The following is a sample of our Patient Information and Admission Booklet

Patient Information and Admission Booklet

Admission Booklet Content

- Introduction
- Agency Information
- Agency Ownership
- Health Team Members
- Office Location
- Medicare and Medicaid Notice
- Notice About Privacy Regarding Outcome & Assessment Information (OASIS)

- Patients Who Do Not Have Medicare or Medicaid Coverage
- Patients Who Do Have Medicare or Medicaid Coverage
- Equipment/Emergency Checklist
- Emergency/Disaster Plan
- Patient's Right to Make Advance Directives
- Notice of Privacy and Confidentiality Practices
- Home Care Patient Rights and Responsibilities
- About The Right To Express Grievances
- Admission Service Agreement
- Patient and Family Education Handouts for:
- Emergency Checklist
- Emergency Management
- Home Safety
- Hazardous Materials and Waste Disposal
- Infection Control
- Oxygen Safety Rules

Introduction

The staff at XYZ Agency appreciates the confidence you have shown in us by allowing us to meet your home healthcare needs. In order that we may serve you in all situations, we have prepared this comprehensive Admission Booklet for you.

Once the Admission process is complete we will make copies of the signed forms for our records. You will be given the original Admission Booklet on or before the day we start services.

Please keep this booklet in a place easily accessible to our staff so they may be better prepared to assist you in the event of an emergency.

Should you have any questions regarding the information contained within this booklet, feel free to call our office.

Sincerely,

Owner/Administrator

Agency Information

Agency Ownership:

XYZ Agency is locally owned and operated by _____.

Health Team Members Names and Position:

Administrator
Director of Clinical Services
Office Manager
Human Resources/Payroll
Clinical Supervisor

Office Location:

XYZ Agency
Street Address
City, State, Zip Code
Telephone Number
Fax Number

XYZ Agency

Notice

XYZ Agency is NOT a Medicare provider. We do not accept Medicare as a payer source.

XYZ Agency is a Medicaid and Medicaid Waiver provider.

XYZ Agency does accept private pay clients.

Acknowledgement:

I have read and understand the above Notice regardless as to my payer source and I request services be provided to me by XYZ Agency.

Client's Signature _____ Date _____

Home Healthcare Representative's Signature and Title

_____

Jeffie Maag

Equipment/Emergency Checklist

Client's Name _____

Medical Record Number _____

Equipment (List type of equipment)

Vendor's Name and Phone Number

Emergency/Disaster Plan

Client's Name _____

Medical Record Number _____

Emergency Plan:

A disaster can occur at any time. Knowing what to do is the best way to be prepared. Due to risks involved, home care visits will be suspended during a disaster and will resume when clearance is issued by the local authorities.

In the event of, but not limited to, a bomb threat, a civil disturbance, or mass casualties such as trauma, disease, hazmat, or terrorist incident, call 911.

In the event of a natural disaster such as a blizzard, earthquake, flooding, hurricane, ice storm, land/mud slide or tornado, take cover in a safe place to protect the patient and yourself. The Safe Place Designated in this home is:

_____

In the event of a communication failure or utility failure call the responsible company.

Phone Company Number _____

Natural Gas Company Number _____

Water Company Number _____

Sewage Company Number _____

Electric Company Number _____

Fire Department call 911

Police Department call 911

Ambulance Services Number _____

In the event you should need to evacuate your home following a disaster, call the American Red Cross for guidance. Phone Number

_____

In the event of a community disaster, turn the TV on Channel _____ or a Radio to _____ for further information.

Client's Signature _____

Date _____

Patient's Right To Make Advance Directives

Please check with your State Department of Health to obtain the appropriate form for your state.

Following the appropriate form and it's completion, we classify each client.

This Patient is Classified as a:

- High Risk
- Medium Risk
- Low Risk

Check the appropriate risk category for this client.

About The Right To Express Grievances

You have the right and responsibility to express concerns, dissatisfaction or make complaints about services you receive or do not receive without fear of reprisal or discrimination. We, at XYZ Agency encourage you to discuss all concerns and complaints with us. The Agency telephone number is _____. When you call, ask to speak with the Director of Clinical Services or the Administrator.

XYZ Agency has a formal grievance procedure that ensures that your concerns shall be reviewed and an investigation started within 48 hours. Every attempt shall be made to resolve all grievances within 14 days. You will be kept informed by telephone of the status of the investigation and may receive a written report when a resolution is determined.

If you feel the need to discuss your concerns, dissatisfaction or complaints with someone other than XYZ Agency staff, the State provides a Home Health "Hot Line". The hours of operation are 8 AM to 4:30 PM and the number is _____.

NOTE TO THE READER:

Check with your state to determine if there is a Home Health "Hot Line" phone number assigned for your state.

Patient and Family Educational Handout

Emergency Management

Always be prepared for a sudden emergency. Be sure to have enough necessities on hand and ask family and/or friends for any help needed.

You may be notified of a possible emergency by weather radio, commercial radio, television stations and/or a door-to-door warning from local emergency officials. Follow their instructions!

Assemble a survival kit which should include the following at a minimum:

- First Aid Kit;
- Three (3) days worth of medications, include a list of the medications you take regularly and their dosages, the name of the physician prescribing them and a list of any allergies to foods and medications;
- If you use insulin, pre-fill syringes for three (3) days;
- If you use medical supplies, have an extra three (3) days of supplies available;
- Have available a list of physicians and relatives/friends who should be notified should you be injured;
- Have available a list of important documents, including any documents for your pets, in a water-proof container;
- Store a flashlight, battery operated radio and extra batteries in case of a power loss;
- Whistle;
- Manual can opener;
- Have cash (including coins) on hand to help you through the emergency period;
- Personal hygiene supplies;
- Hand sanitizer; and
- Insurance Agent's name and telephone number.

If you use oxygen, arrange for a back-up unit.

If you have an intravenous site you will need extra sterile water to clean the IV site.

Store three (3) days worth of non-perishable food and water; you will need one (1) gallon of water per day per person.

Store a change of clothing and a blanket or sleeping bag in a watertight plastic bag.

Keep your supplies packed and ready in one place before an emergency/natural disaster strikes. Be sure the container that you put your emergency supplies into has an ID tag or is marked to identify what it is.

When an emergency/natural disaster occurs, it is always best to be prepared and take extra steps to make an already bad situation less stressful. Other things to consider are:

- Label any equipment, such as wheelchairs, canes or walkers.
- Arrange for a back-up power source for any medical equipment that operates on electricity.
- Make arrangements to stay with relatives or friends in the event of an emergency.
- If necessary, make arrangements in advance for special transportation and/or stay at a shelter.

If you are told to stay indoors due to bad weather:

- Close all windows and doors in your home.
- Turn off all fans, heating and air conditioning systems as needed.
- Go to a room with the fewest windows and doors.
- Stay away from all windows to avoid injury from flying glass and/or other projectiles.

If you are instructed to evacuate your home:

- Call the home health agency and give the address and telephone number where you can be reached.
- Turn off all electricity and water before leaving your home.
- Leave immediately, even if the weather is nice.

- Stay away from any electrical wires.
- Remember to lock your windows and doors when you evacuate your home.

Please be aware that during an emergency the home health agency personnel will NOT be providing services in areas that have been designated unsafe!

Patient and Family Educational Handout

Home Safety

You can protect yourself and/or your caregiver from injuries or accidents while in your home.

General Safety Tips

- Keep all emergency numbers by your telephone.
- Avoid wearing only socks, smooth-soled shoes or slippers on uncarpeted floors.
- Avoid wet floors; wipe up spills immediately.
- Keep a clear path through your home. Move objects that could trip you, like electrical cords or throw rugs.
- Be sure you have enough light to see where you are walking. Keep a night light on or keep a flashlight by your bed.
- Keep all of your supplies and medication out of reach of children.
- If you are using medical electrical equipment and your home does not have three-pronged outlets, use a three-pronged adapter. For safe use of the adapter, securely attach the green wire to the center screw of the outlet cover plate.

Medication Safety

- Tell your physician, pharmacist and nurse about all the medications you are taking (both prescription and over-the-counter).
- Remember to tell the home health nurse if any of your medications change.

- Throw away any expired medications.
- Never take someone else's medications.

Disposal Tips

- If you have procedures that requires needles, DO NOT recap your needles. To prevent accidental needle sticks to yourself and/or others, all used needles and syringes should be dispose of in an approved safety container.
- If you are receiving chemotherapy at home, all used chemotherapy drugs and supplies should be disposed of in an approved safety container.
- If you have soiled dressings, disposable sheets and/or medical gloves, place them in securely fastened plastic bags before you put them in the garbage can with your other trash.

Fire Safety

- Make sure fire exits are free of clutter so you can get out should a fire occur.
- Make sure your smoke/fire detectors are in good working order.
- Never smoke or let others smoke while oxygen is in use.
- Never smoke or let others smoke around oxygen containers.
- Keep a fire extinguisher handy and learn how to use it.
- Don't smoke in bed, or if you are feeling sleepy.
- Keep all electrical appliances in good working order.
- Call your home health agency should you have any additional safety questions.

Patient and Family Educational Handout

Hazardous Materials and Waste Disposal

Proper disposal of waste in the home will insure safety and infection control for you and others, such as your family.

Please follow these steps:

- Always wear disposable gloves when handling blood, body fluids or body waste.
- Wash any surfaces or equipment that have been contaminated with blood, other body fluids or body waste. Wash area with soap and water, then clean with diluted household bleach (10 part water to 1 part bleach). Use paper towels - not reusable sponges. Always wear disposable gloves. Put disposable items into a plastic-lined bag, then in another garbage bag. Remove gloves, making sure you do not touch the outside of the gloves with your bare hands and discard them into the second garbage bag. Be sure all bags are closed securely and discard it into a trash can with a tight fitting lid.
- Put all needles, syringes and related equipment in a puncture-resistant safety container or sharps container. Needles should not be recapped, bent, broken, removed from syringes or otherwise handled. Place the safety/sharps container in a garbage bag and then into a trash can with a tight fitting lid. Follow local laws and regulations for disposal of used safety/sharps containers.
- Carefully pour blood and body waste down the drain to avoid splashing, or flush down a toilet connected to a sanitary sewage system. (In rural areas, consult your County Health Department for proper disposal).
- Put tissues, soiled dressing, used tampons, sanitary pads and diapers into a plastic-lined bag. This bag should be placed in another garbage bag and then placed into a trash can with a tight fitting lid. Follow local Regulations for solid waste management.

- Put chemotherapy waste (needles, syringes, used container, and IV tubing) in a puncture-resistant "Chemotherapy Container". Place this safety container in a garbage bag and then into a trash can with a tight fitting lid. Dispose of chemotherapy waste according to local regulations for solid waste management.
- Medical waste may require special pick-up in your area. Check with your local city government for further information and instructions on proper disposal.

Patient and Family Educational Handout

Infection Control

If you have any of the following signs of infection, call your physician right away:

- Rise in body temperature above 100 degrees F.
- Tenderness, pain, swelling, redness, or drainage around a catheter site, wound(s), or tubes.
- Rashes, spots or other skin disorders.
- Immobility.

To reduce the risk of infection, please follow these guidelines:

- Wash hand before and after each patient contact or procedure.
- Always wear gloves when handling blood or body fluids, or when in contact with mucous membranes or open cuts.
- Any caregiver with an open cut or other skin condition should not care for the patient.
- Never re-cap needles. Always dispose of needles in a safety container.
- Use only disposable razors for shaving.
- No one else should use the patient's thermometer.
- Wash dirty dishes in detergent and hot water right away.
- Avoid contact with anyone who has a cold or infectious disease. If your caregiver has a cold or flu symptoms, he/she should wear a mask.
- Daily personal cleanliness is very important.
- Keep soiled sheets, towel and clothing in a container lined with a plastic bag until laundered. Laundry should be done in hot water.
- Change dressing and do catheter care as scheduled or as directed by your physician or nurse.
- Limit contact with pets.

- Wash surfaces or equipment, contaminated with blood or other body fluids, with a solution of detergent, water and diluted household bleach (10 parts water to 1 part bleach).
- Throw out patient's leftover portions of food right away.

Patient and Family Educational Handout

Oxygen Safety Rules

Oxygen does not explode. Oxygen does not burn by itself, but it is one (1) of the three (3) ingredients necessary for a fire to occur. The other two (2) ingredients are a combustible or flammable material and a source of ignition. To prevent the chance of fire, follow these rules:

Do Not

- Do not permit the use of open flames or burning tobacco in the room where oxygen is being used or stored.
- Do not use any household electric equipment in an oxygen enriched atmosphere (i.e., electric razors, heaters and blankets). Keep these type of items at least five (5) feet from oxygen.
- Do not use aerosol sprays in the vicinity of oxygen equipment.
- Do not oil or grease oxygen equipment.
- Do not allow oxygen "on" when equipment is not in use.
- Do not allow oxygen tubing to be covered by any objects.
- Do not use or handle oxygen containers roughly.
- Do not store oxygen in a confined area.
- Do not allow untrained persons to use or adjust any oxygen equipment.
- Do not attempt to fix or repair oxygen equipment.
- Do not store oxygen containers near radiators, heat ducts, steam pipes or other sources of heat.
- Do not open cylinder valves quickly.
- Do not remove oxygen tanks from stand.
- Do not transport oxygen in an enclosed area or the trunk of your car.
- Do not alter the liter flow from what your physician prescribes.

Do's

- It is advisable to have "NO SMOKING" signs visible throughout the home.
- Consider having fire extinguishers available.
- Do transport portable oxygen tanks in the back seat of your car and secure it tightly
- Do open your window approximately one (1) inch when transporting any oxygen equipment.

Jeffie Maag

ADMISSION SERVICE AGREEMENT
For
XYZ Agency

CONSENT FOR CARE/SERVICE

I hereby consent and authorize the agency, its agents and associates to provide care and treatment to me in my home as prescribed by my physician and per program policy. I understand that I must have an attending physician at all times for the duration of this agreement, unless the organization determines otherwise. I have received an explanation of the services to be provided (including disciplines, proposed frequency of visits and anticipated outcomes), my involvement with the plan of care, and how changes will be made if needed. I understand that I and/or my family/caregiver will be responsible for my care in the absence of the agency staff.

AUTHORIZATION FOR RELEASE OF INFORMATION

I hereby consent to and authorize the agency to release and receive information for the purpose of treatment, payment and health care operations. The exchange of information may occur between, but is not limited to: physicians, third party payers, other health care providers, and regulatory and/or crediting reviewers.

LIABILITY FOR PAYMENT

I certify that all the information given by me to the agency is correct for requesting and applying for payment under Title XVIII (Medicare), Title XIX (Medicaid) of the Social Security Act and/or from any third party payer. I understand and agree to pay deductibles, co-payments, spend downs and any amount due after payment of benefits on my behalf by any and all third party payers.

- I verify that I am
- I verify that I am not

A participating member of an HMO (Health Maintenance Organization). If I enroll in one I will immediately notify the agency.

I understand that services provided to me XYZ Agency will be billed as follows:

- Medicare fee for services (Projected 100% covered).
- Medicaid (Projected 100% covered after meeting spend down and/or other requirements by Medicaid.)
- Insurance coverage varies with each individual policy. The patient's anticipated payment amounts per visit will be provided in writing when the insurance company informs the agency of the patient's financial liability. When know at time of Admission: Projected _____% of charges to be covered after deductible is met.
- Private Pay at $_____ per hour. Patient is responsible for the timely payment.

ASSIGNMENT OF BENEFITS

I request that payment of authorized benefits be made on my behalf directly to the agency.

This Admission Agreement is applicable to this admission to XYZ Agency. I understand what I have read and what was explained to me and I agree to the terms and conditions as stated above. Additionally, I understand that either party may terminate this agreement for any reason and/or at any time.

Anticipated hours for Skilled Nursing is _____ hours, _____ times per week and or Respite Care for an average of _____ hours per month.

I acknowledge that I have read, understand and agree to the terms of this Admission Agreement.

Patient or Authorized Representative Signature _____
If signed by other than the client, state relationship _____

Jeffie Maag

Agency Representative Signature Date _____
Client's Name   Medical Record Number _____

There a number of Admission Agreement forms available online and from MCN Library.

Admission Acknowledgment Form

Patient's Name _____MR#_____

I acknowledge that the following information has been provided to me and reviewed with me by a member of the home health agency.

Patient to initial each box regarding the Admission Booklet with the following information:

- Agency Ownership
- Health Team Members
- Office Address
- Medicare/Medicaid Notice
- Collection of Information (OASIS)
- Medicare/Medicaid & Private Pay
- Equipment/Emergency Checklist
- Equipment/Disaster Plan
- Advance Directives
- Notice of Privacy and Confidentiality Practices
- Home Care Patient Rights and Responsibilities
- About The Right To Express Grievances
- Patient and Family Educational Handouts
- Admission Service Agreement
- Plan of Care
- Other

Patient's Signature _____Date _____
If signed other than the patient state relationship _____
Agency Representative Signature and Title _____

CHAPTER 23

Insurance Coverage

I recommend you start working with an insurance agent on getting the best price for insurance as soon as possible. You will need to have the following types of insurance coverage:

- Unemployment Insurance
- Workers Compensation Insurance
- General Liability Insurance
- Malpractice and Professional Liability Insurance.

Your insurance agent should be knowledgeable in knowing how much coverage you will be required to have in your specific state. I, for one, like working with a local agent who I can see face-to-face when I have questions.

CHAPTER 24

Payroll and Accounting Services

There are a number of payroll companies out there. You should research each company because there are costs involved, and unless you intend to do your own payroll, you will want to get the biggest bang for your buck.

Do not be afraid to negotiate for the best possible deal. Every penny counts when it's your business.

The accounting firm you intend to use may have an in-house payroll processing division. Your large national payroll companies offer a lot of different services but you will have to pay for them.

You will need to develop an operating budget and a capital budget. Keep in mind that you are in the process of opening a new business, and that your expenses will be greater than they will be in the coming years. A budget should be realistic and factual. Be sure to keep all receipts for tax purposes.

Our agency uses Quick Books for our accounting system. It is compatible with most payroll and accounting firms you will be working with.

CHAPTER 25

Medical Director

Now is the time to forge ahead and find a doctor who is willing to serve as your agency Medical Director. The nice thing about getting a Medical Director for home health care is you reimburse him/her for the actual time spent working with your agency. This is different from long term care where you pay a flat monthly rate.

You can find a number of free Medical Director Agreement templates on-line that you can use for your agency.

CHAPTER 26

OIG Exclusion List

Every employee and vendor you use must be checked against the OIG Exclusion List. I recommend you recheck every employee and vendor against the OIG Exclusion List every three (3) months.

I recommend you take the time to go on-line to the Office of the Inspector General and read about the exclusion list.

CHAPTER 27

Meeting Your Local Caseworkers

Now is the time to get your company name out there. You need to share with anyone and everyone what it is you are going to be doing, the type of clients you intend to take care of, and how far along you are in the start-up process.

The case workers at your local Family and Children Services can be very helpful in sharing information about who within their organization handles Medicaid clients and types of waiver programs available within your area.

Hospital discharge planners are another resource you need to make contact with and set up a time to meet with them to share what services your home health agency will be providing.

Don't be afraid to ask questions and share with the world what you are doing.

CHAPTER 28

Getting Your Sampling Clients

Trying to get the sampling clients we needed for the "pro bono" requirement was very difficult. The elderly or disabled are suspicious of a company that offers to provide a service to them at no charge for a period of six to eight weeks. What I found to be the best and easiest way to get our sampling clients was to go to a low income high rise apartment complex and talk with the social worker or apartment manager about what I needed to do.

We explained to the case worker that we were opening up a new home health care agency, and in order for us to be surveyed by the state we had to take on ten "pro bono" clients for a period of six to eight weeks, and during this time we would be surveyed by our State Department of Health to determine if we were competent as nurses and as an agency to be licensed. We went on to explain that this service was at no cost to the clients or housing complex but that there were certain requirements that had to be met by those we would provide care to. We explained that the clients would have to be considered "home bound" and need some type of skilled service. We asked the social worker if she could pick out clients that would benefit from Diabetic Management, Medication Management, Falls Risk Management and/or Wound Management. To our surprise within a week we had clients lined up that fell into every category.

CHAPTER 29

Final Review

By now you must be starting to wonder, "Will I ever get this agency opened?" If everything is in place you need to take a deep breath because the next step will require a lot of attention. I recommend you do a double check to make sure you have not missed one thing. If you find everything is in place, then it is time to move forward.

Now that we had our sampling we submitted our paper work to request a Probationary License from our State Department of Health Home Health Care Division. Within a week we had our letter of approval. This was an exciting time for us and we wanted to make sure we did everything right the first time around.

Your Probationary License is good for six months. The letter you receive from your Department of Health will have instructions on how to access the OASIS web site. Be sure to keep this information safeguarded.

The OASIS web interchange is where you input information into the computer on most clients that receive care from your agency. The OASIS is a standardized form that is used to do an assessment on a client.

Every state may have difference requirements, so make sure you know what it is they expect from your agency.

CHAPTER 30

Admitting The Clients

Now that you have your Probationary License it is time to start the admitting process. Contact the social worker you have been working with regarding your client sampling and set up a date and time to meet each client to conduct the assessment and put him/her on case load. Before actually assessing the client you need to make sure you have a physician's order to assess for home health care and to provided skilled nursing. Your first client once assessed and admitted by an RN, his/her information will be used for input into the OASIS computerized system as your trial client. The information the RN will be putting in the computer for the first time will demonstrate the RN's ability to input information into the OASIS system correctly. Whatever you do, just make sure you follow the instructions sent to you by your State Department of Health, Home Health Care Division.

Our state required we input only one client into the OASIS system but every client was required to have a comprehensive assessment done. As each client is admitted and assessed, the RN will need to complete a Plan Of Care on the Client and a Prior Authorization. Both of these forms will be required to be signed by the client's individual attending physician. If this client was not a "pro bono" case you would submit the Plan of Care and Prior Authorization to the appropriate insurance carrier for approval.

The RN will need to create a Medication Profile, Medication Administration Record and any teaching tools needed.

As you see, the admitting process is very time consuming and you can not afford to make any mistakes at this point. I recommend you only admit one to two clients a week unless you have several RN's working for you.

CHAPTER 31

Survey Readiness

By this time you have admitted ten clients and have completed all the paper work and seen each one of the clients at least once. Your state may require that you have several discharged clients as well. Now you are ready to submit your request to have the initial survey conducted on your agency. Since the survey is unannounced, all I can say is just be ready.

The surveyor will want to go into several client homes and watch the nurse perform services as outlined on the client's Plan of Care. Once the surveyor gives you the names of the clients she wants to see, call the clients and let them know the survey is taking place and that the surveyor wants to visit them. Keep in mind that the same nurse for one client can not be the nurse for the other clients in the sampling. The surveyor will most likely want to visit at least three clients.

With all the hard work you and your team have put into getting your agency up and running, you will hopefully pass your survey the first time around. Remember, organization counts.

Once the survey process is over you will need to do discharge planning on each of the clients.

CHAPTER 32

Getting Credentialed For Funding

Our agency chose not to take Medicare clients. We primarily wanted to deal with children so we decided on Medicaid (state funding) and private pay clients. I contacted the Director of Medicaid at the state level for an application. Once I received the application, I looked it over and it looked simple enough, so I filled it out and submitted it, not once, but twice. Both times it was declined. All it takes is one simple mistake on the application and then it is archived.

I then talked with a Nurse Practitioner who gave me the name of an individual who did credentialing for doctors and therapist. I made an appointment and met with her. She got the application approved the first time around. It was worth the money spent to get my Medicaid funding approved. In my state there are several divisions within Medicaid, and each division requires separate credentialing, and she was able to accomplish this for my agency. Once this was achieved we were ready to start admitting and gladly accept payment for our services.

It took us about 9 months to get to this point and had I of had the information in this book I could have reduced that time frame to about 4 months.

Jeffie Maag

Some insurance companies may require additional credentialing through organizations such as, JACHO or CHAP. To obtain this credentialing cost a lot of money but opens doors of opportunity if you want to work with insurance companies.

Once all the credentialing is done, you will need to set up the programs for billing. Check with your state as to which form is required for the various types of billing. Your state may assist you by providing training regarding the billing process.

Be sure to utilize your state's director at the Department of Health for Home Health Care. He or she can answer questions or direct you to the manuals needed. Most manuals required are on the state's web site and can be printed. I suggest you read the manuals before printing, because not all of the information in the manual will pertain to home health care. Print off what you need and download the rest to your computer.

CHAPTER 33

In Closing

This program is not for everyone, but if this is what you want to do, you will find this information very helpful.

I am sure I did not cover everything, but I can assure you that I have covered a lot of information that was not offered to me. I had to do months and months of research to get my agency opened.

It takes a lot of preparation to get a business up and running, so don't get discouraged. The end will be in sight before you know it. I grew my agency slowly so issues we encountered could be fixed before they got out of control. Also, we were able to hire the right person for each client, because of the waiting period from the time we accepted a client to the approval process.

I truly wish you the very best in making your dream a reality. I know if I could do it on my own then you can do it with the information I have provided.

www.ingramcontent.com/pod-product-compliance
Lightning Source LLC
Chambersburg PA
CBHW021009180526
45163CB00005B/1947